BREAST CANCER DIET COOKBOOK FOR NEWLY DIAGNOSED 2024

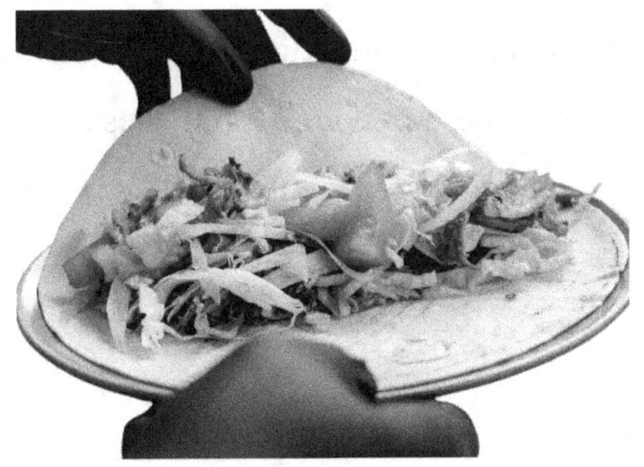

Transform daily meals into moments of self-care, promoting physical and emotional healing.

Misty J Font

TABLE OF CONTENT

CHAPTER 4 : DESSERTS AND TREATS 45

CHAPTER 5: SNACK ATTACKS............... 55

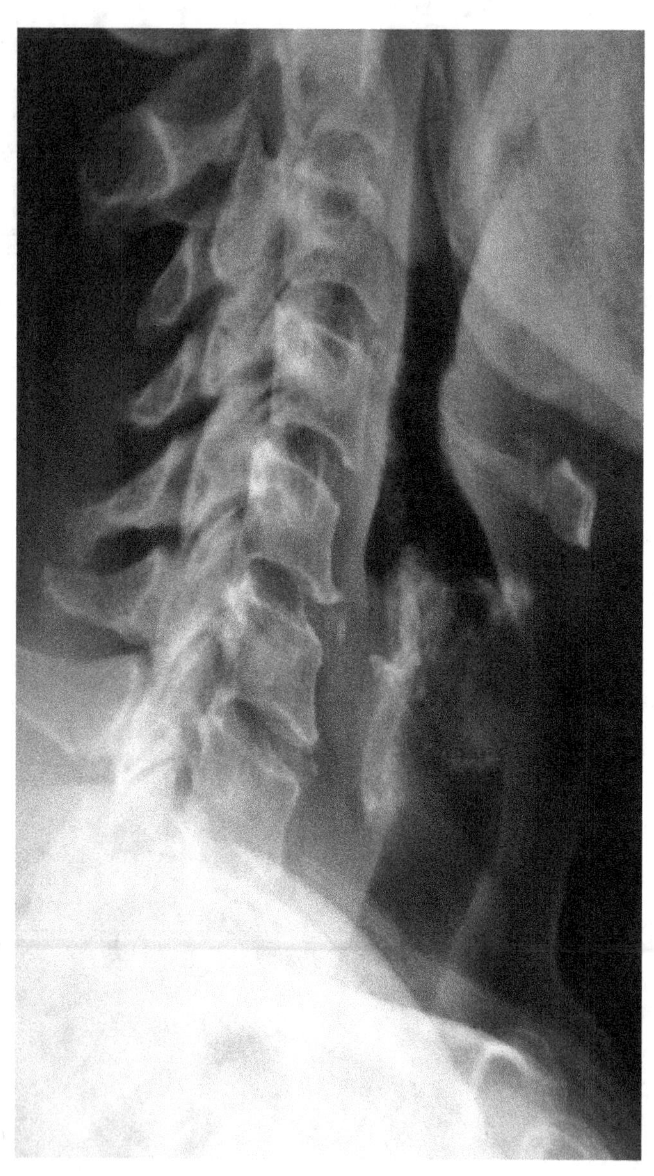

INTRODUCTION

Grace's battle with breast cancer was not only a story of tenacity, but also a testament to the healing power of mindful nutrition. When she received her diagnosis, she was determined to approach her treatment holistically, incorporating dietary choices that complemented her medical plan.

Grace discovered a Breast Cancer Diet Cookbook in her search for a nourishing and supportive diet, and it became her guide to recovery. This cookbook was more than just a collection of recipes; it was a well-researched resource tailored to the nutritional needs of breast cancer patients. It became an indispensable tool in Grace's healing journey, filled with expert advice and recipes chosen for their potential health benefits.

Grace used the cookbook to guide her through a plethora of recipes designed to provide essential nutrients, support immune function, and promote overall well-being during her treatment. From anti-inflammatory breakfasts to antioxidant-rich snacks, the cookbook provided a diverse range of options that made her daily meals not only nourishing but also enjoyable.

Grace's favourite recipe was Turmeric Lentil Soup, a hearty bowl of ingredients known for their anti-cancer properties. She found solace in the Golden Milk Turmeric Latte, a warm and soothing drink that became a nightly ritual for her. These recipes, rooted in both flavour and nutritional wisdom, not only aided her physical recovery but also lifted her spirits during difficult times.

Grace's journey was more than just following a recipe; it was a comprehensive approach to self-care. The cookbook enabled her to make informed food choices, giving her a sense of control and agency in her healing process. Grace discovered not only a path to physical recovery but also a renewed connection to her own well-being as she embraced the nourishing power of the Breast Cancer Diet Cookbook. Her story serves as a beacon of hope for others facing similar challenges, demonstrating how mindful nutrition can play an important role in the road to recovery and resilience.

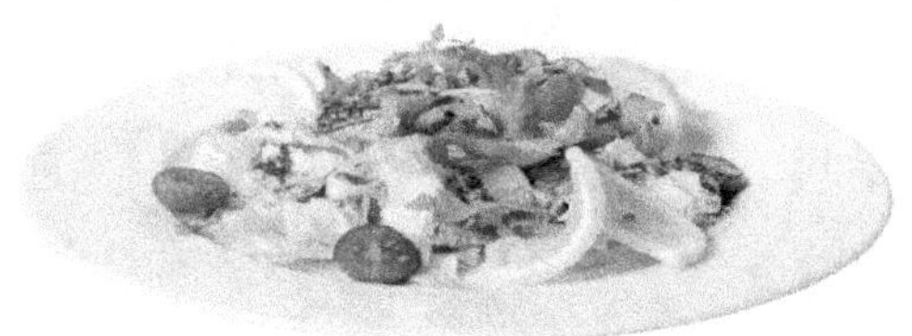

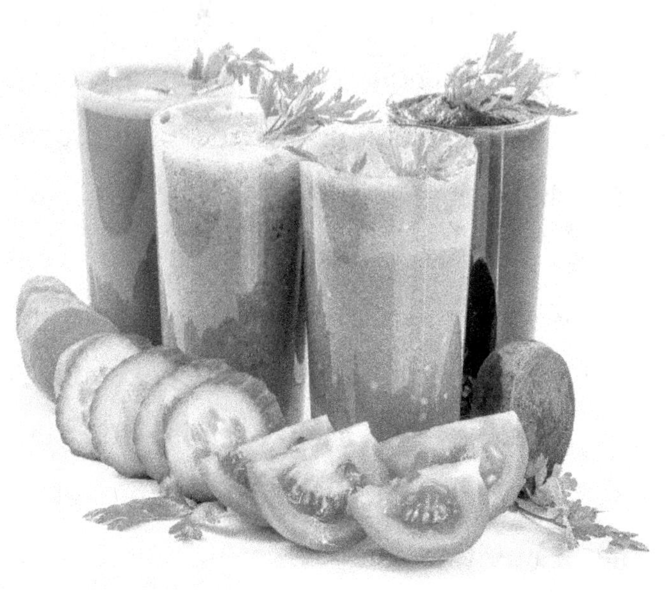

CHAPTER 1: BREAKFASTS

Quinoa Breakfast Bowl

Ingredients:

- Quinoa
- Almond milk
- Fresh berries
- Chia seeds

Instructions:

1. Cook the quinoa according to the package directions.
2. Combine with almond milk and serve with fresh berries and chia seeds on top.

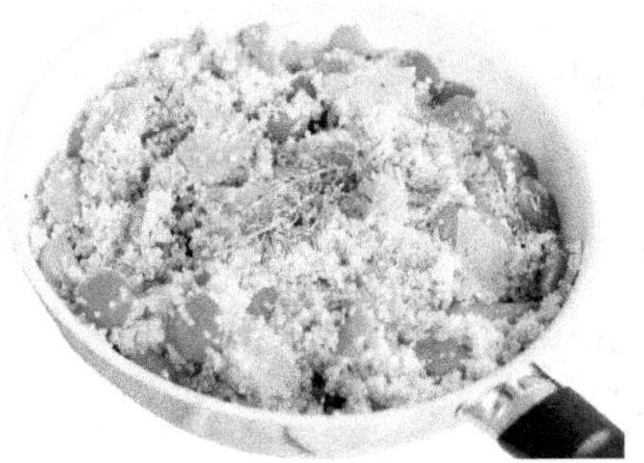

Avocado Toast with Smoked Salmon

Ingredients:

- Whole-grain bread
- Avocado
- Smoked salmon
- Lemon juice

Instructions:

1. Toast the bread.
2. Spread avocado on bread.
3. Serve with smoked salmon and lemon juice on top.

Greek Yogurt Parfait

Ingredients:

- Greek yogurt
- Granola
- Mixed berries
- Honey

Instructions:

1. Layer Greek yoghurt, granola, and berries on a plate.
2. Drizzle with honey to finish.

Egg White Veggie Omelette

Ingredients:

- Egg whites
- Spinach
- Tomatoes
- Mushrooms

Instructions:

1. Pour egg whites into a pan after whisking them.
2. Mix in the spinach, tomatoes, and mushrooms.
3. Cook until the mixture is firm.

Chia Seed Pudding

Ingredients:

- Chia seeds
- Almond milk
- Vanilla extract
- Sliced almonds

Instructions:

1. Combine the chia seeds, almond milk, and vanilla essence in a mixing bowl.
2. Refrigerate for at least 24 hours.
3. Serve with sliced almonds on top.

Turmeric Smoothie

Ingredients:

- Banana
- Pineapple
- Turmeric
- Almond milk

Instructions:

1. Blend the banana, pineapple, turmeric,

2. and almond milk together.

Sweet Potato Breakfast Hash

Ingredients:

- Sweet potatoes
- Red bell pepper
- Onion
- Olive oil

Instructions:

- Cut the sweet potatoes, pepper, and onion into dice.
- Cook in olive oil until done.

Salmon and Asparagus Frittata

Ingredients:

- Eggs
- Smoked salmon

* Asparagus

* Dill

Instructions:

1. Whisk the eggs and place them into a pan.

2. Serve with smoked salmon, asparagus, and dill.

3. Bake until the cheese has melted.

Blueberry Almond Muffins

Ingredients:

* Almond flour

* Blueberries

* Greek yogurt

* Baking soda

Instructions:

1. Combine almond flour, blueberries, Greek yoghurt, and baking soda in a mixing bowl.

2. Make muffins.

Coconut and Berry Smoothie Bowl

Ingredients:

- Coconut milk
- Mixed berries
- Shredded coconut
- Granola

Instructions:

1. Blend the coconut milk and fruit together.
2. Top with granola and shredded coconut.

Spinach and Mushroom Breakfast Wrap

Ingredients:

- Whole-grain wrap
- Spinach

- Mushrooms

- Feta cheese

Instructions:

1. Sauté the spinach and mushrooms before filling the wrap.

2. Roll it up with the feta cheese on top.

Cauliflower Breakfast Bowl

Ingredients:

- Cauliflower rice

- Broccoli

- Cherry tomatoes

- Poached egg

Instructions:

1. Cauliflower rice, broccoli, and cherry tomatoes should be sautéed.

2. Serve with a poached egg on top.

Pumpkin Spice Overnight Oats

Ingredients:

- Rolled oats
- Pumpkin puree
- Cinnamon
- Maple syrup

Instructions:

1. Combine oats, pumpkin puree, cinnamon, and maple syrup in a mixing bowl.
2. Refrigerate for at least 24 hours.

Almond Butter and Banana Smoothie

Ingredients:

- Almond butter
- Banana
- Almond milk
- Ice

Instructions:

1. Blend together the almond butter, banana, almond milk,
2. and ice.

Tomato and Basil Breakfast Quiche

Ingredients:

- Eggs
- Tomatoes
- Fresh basil
- Mozzarella cheese

Instructions:

1. Whisk the eggs together and pour into a pie plate.
2. Sliced tomatoes, fresh basil, and mozzarella are optional.
3. Bake until the cheese has melted.

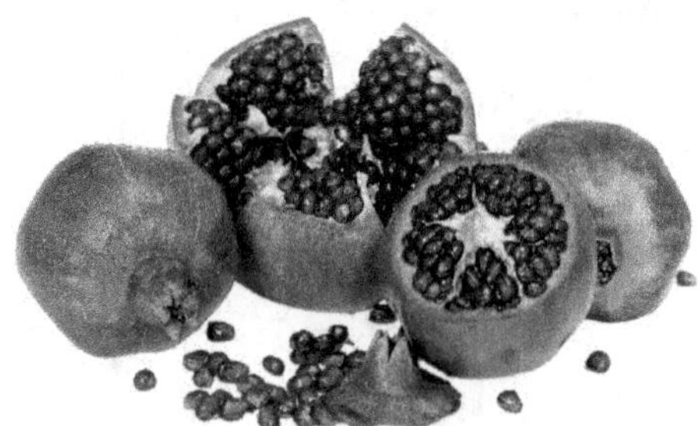

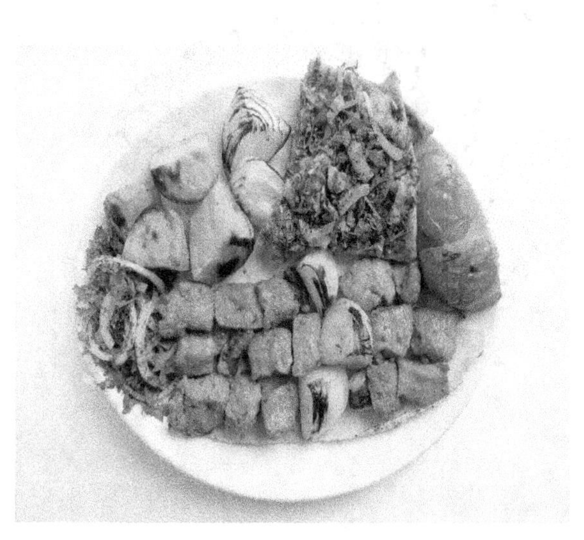

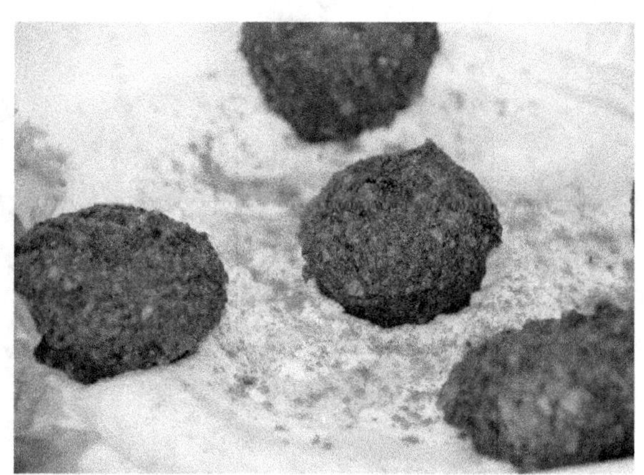

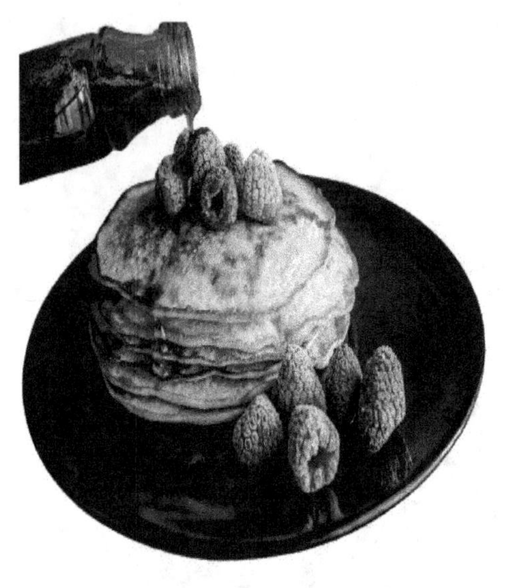

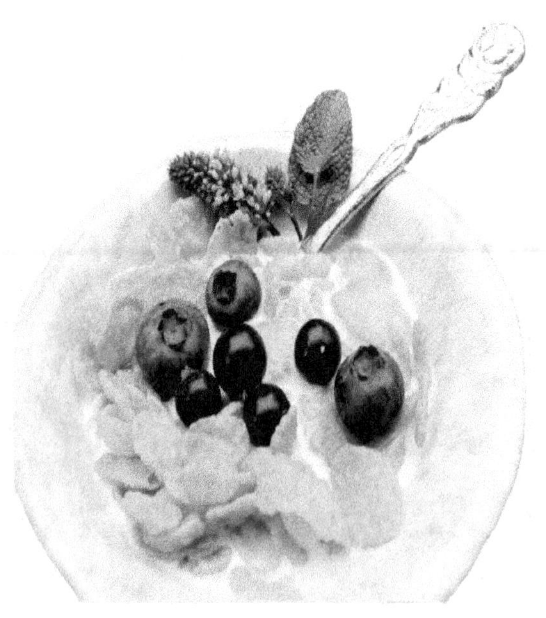

CHAPTER 2: LUNCH

Grilled Lemon Herb Chicken Salad

Ingredients:

- Chicken breast
- Mixed greens
- Cherry tomatoes
- Lemon

Instructions:

1. Lemon and herb-grilled chicken.
2. Toss with mixed greens and cherry tomatoes before serving.

Quinoa and Black Bean Bowl

Ingredients:

- Quinoa
- Black beans
- Avocado
- Lime

Instructions:

1. Cook the quinoa and combine it with the black beans.
2. Top with avocado slices and a squeeze of lime.

Salmon and Vegetable Stir-Fry

Ingredients:

- Salmon fillet
- Broccoli
- Bell peppers
- Low-sodium soy sauce

Instructions:

1. Stir-fry fish, broccoli,
2. and bell peppers in low-sodium soy sauce.

Mushroom and Spinach Stuffed Bell Peppers

Ingredients:

- Bell peppers
- Mushrooms
- Spinach
- Quinoa

Instructions:

1. Sauté the mushrooms and spinach together. Combine with the cooked quinoa.
2. Bake until the bell peppers are soft.

Turmeric Lentil Soup

Ingredients:

- Red lentils
- Carrots
- Turmeric
- Vegetable broth

Instructions:

1. Sauté the mushrooms and spinach together.
2. Combine with the cooked quinoa.
3. Bake until the bell peppers are soft.

Cabbage and Chickpea Salad

Ingredients:

- Shredded cabbage
- Chickpeas
- Cucumber
- Olive oil

Instructions:

- Toss together the shredded cabbage, chickpeas, and cucumber.
- Dress with olive oil.

Lemon Garlic Shrimp Skewers

Ingredients:

- Shrimp
- Garlic
- Lemon
- Olive oil

Instructions:

1. Garlic, lemon and olive oil marinate the prawns.
2. Grill and skewer.

Sweet Potato and Kale Salad

Ingredients:

- Sweet potatoes
- Kale
- Pomegranate seeds
- Balsamic vinaigrette

Instructions:

1. Toss roasted sweet potatoes with spinach and pomegranate seeds.
2. Drizzle with balsamic vinaigrette and serve.

Cauliflower and Broccoli Soup

Ingredients:

- Cauliflower
- Broccoli
- Onion
- Almond milk

Instructions:

1. Cook cauliflower, broccoli, and onion in almond milk.
2. Blend until completely smooth.

Greek Chicken Wrap

Ingredients:

- Grilled chicken strips
- Whole-grain wrap
- Greek yogurt
- Cucumber

Instructions:

1. Wrap grilled chicken, Greek yoghurt,
2. and cucumber in a wrap.

Sesame Ginger Tofu Stir-Fry

Ingredients:

- Tofu
- Broccoli
- Snow peas
- Sesame ginger sauce

Instructions:

- Tofu, broccoli, and snow peas in a sesame ginger sauce.

Roasted Vegetable Quinoa Bowl

Ingredients:

- Roasted vegetables (zucchini, bell peppers, carrots)
- Quinoa
- Feta cheese
- Lemon vinaigrette

Instructions:

1. Combine roasted veggies, quinoa, and feta cheese in a mixing bowl.
2. Dress with the lemon vinaigrette.

Caprese Salad with Grilled Chicken

Ingredients:

- Grilled chicken
- Tomatoes
- Fresh mozzarella
- Basil

Instructions:

1. Combine roasted veggies, quinoa, and feta cheese in a mixing bowl.

2. Dress with the lemon vinaigrette.

Broccoli and Salmon Quiche

Ingredients:

- Broccoli
- Smoked salmon
- Eggs
- Almond flour crust

Instructions:

1. Mix broccoli, smoked salmon, and eggs.

2. Fill an almond flour crust with the mixture.

3. Bake until the cheese has melted.

Lentil and Vegetable Wrap

Ingredients:

- Cooked lentils

- Mixed vegetables (bell peppers, onions, carrots)

- Whole-grain wrap

- Hummus

Instructions:

1. Sauté the veggies and combine them with the lentils.

2. Wrap the mixture and hummus in a wrap.

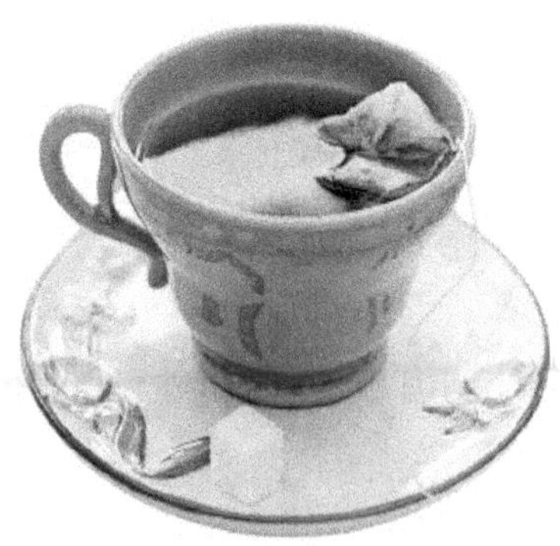

CHAPTER 3 : DINNER

Baked Lemon Garlic Salmon

Ingredients:

- Salmon fillets
- Garlic
- Lemon
- Fresh herbs (such as dill or parsley)

Instructions:

1. On a baking sheet, place the salmon fillets.
2. Rub with garlic powder, lemon juice, and fresh herbs.
3. Bake until the fish is fully done.

Vegetarian Quinoa Stuffed Bell Peppers

Ingredients:

- Bell peppers
- Quinoa
- Black beans
- Corn

Instructions:

1. Cook the quinoa and combine it with the black beans and corn.
2. Bake until the bell peppers are soft.

Herb Grilled Chicken Breast

Ingredients:

- Chicken breast
- Olive oil
- Mixed herbs (rosemary, thyme, oregano)
- Lemon

Instructions:

1. Marinate the chicken in olive oil, herbs, and lemon juice for 30 minutes.
2. Grill until well cooked.

Spaghetti Squash with Tomato Basil Sauce

Ingredients:

- Spaghetti squash
- Tomatoes
- Garlic
- Basil

Instructions:

1. Roast spaghetti squash with a fresh tomato and
2. basil sauce on top.

Turmeric and Ginger Stir-Fried Tofu

Ingredients:

- Tofu
- Turmeric

- Ginger
- Mixed vegetables

Instructions:

1. Tofu, turmeric, ginger,
2. and assorted veggies are stir-fried.

Mushroom and Spinach Quinoa Risotto

Ingredients:

- Quinoa
- Mushrooms
- Spinach
- Vegetable broth

Instructions:

1. Cook quinoa with mushrooms, spinach,
2. and vegetable broth.

Grilled Vegetable and Chicken Kabobs

Ingredients:

- Chicken chunks
- Zucchini
- Cherry tomatoes
- Bell peppers

Instructions:

1. Skewer the chicken and veggies.
2. Grill the chicken and veggies until done.

Cauliflower Rice Stir-Fry with Shrimp

Ingredients:

- Cauliflower rice
- Shrimp
- Broccoli
- Soy sauce

Instructions:

1. Cauliflower rice, prawns, broccoli
2. and soy sauce stir-fry.

Baked Sweet Potato with Chickpea and Spinach

Ingredients:

- Sweet potatoes
- Chickpeas
- Spinach
- Cumin

Instructions:

1. Bake sweet potatoes.
2. Top with a chickpea, spinach, and cumin mixture.

Lemon Herb Baked Chicken Thighs

Ingredients:

- Chicken thighs

- Lemon

- Herbs (thyme, rosemary)

- Olive oil

Instructions:

1. Marinate chicken thighs in lemon, herbs, and olive oil for 30 minutes.

2. Bake until well done.

Eggplant and Tomato Gratin

Ingredients:

- Eggplant

- Tomatoes

- Garlic

- Parmesan cheese

Instructions:

1. In a baking dish, layer sliced eggplant and tomatoes,

2. then top with minced garlic and Parmesan cheese and bake until bubbling.

Sesame-Crusted Tuna Steak

Ingredients:

- Tuna steaks
- Sesame seeds
- Soy sauce
- Ginger

Instructions:

1. Coat tuna steaks in sesame seeds.
2. Sear with soy sauce and ginger in a pan.

Roasted Brussels Sprouts and Chicken Thighs

Ingredients:

- Chicken thighs

- Brussels sprouts
- Olive oil
- Balsamic vinegar

Instructions:

1. Toss together the chicken thighs and Brussels sprouts with the olive oil and balsamic vinegar.
2. Cook until the potatoes are golden brown.

Baked Cod with Lemon Dill Sauce

Ingredients:

- Cod fillets
- Lemon
- Fresh dill
- Greek yogurt

Instructions:

1. In a baking dish, place the fish fillets.

2. For the sauce, combine lemon, dill, and Greek yoghurt.

3. Bake until the fish is tender.

Lentil and Vegetable Curry

Ingredients:

- Lentils
- Mixed vegetables (carrots, peas, bell peppers)
- Curry spices
- Coconut milk

Instructions:

1. In a curry sauce with coconut milk, cook lentils

2. and mixed veggies.

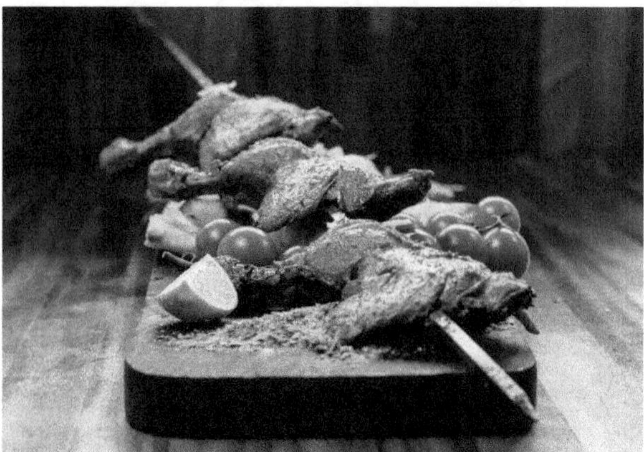

CHAPTER 4 : DESSERTS AND TREATS

Chia Seed Pudding with Berries

Ingredients:

- Chia seeds
- Almond milk
- Fresh berries
- Honey

Instructions:

1. Chia seeds and almond milk should be mixed together.
2. Refrigerate until completely set.
3. Drizzle with honey and top with fresh berries.

Baked Apples with Cinnamon

Ingredients:

- Apples

- Cinnamon

- Walnuts

- Greek yogurt

Instructions:

1. Remove the cores from the apples and sprinkle with cinnamon.

2. Bake until the potatoes are soft.

3. Add crumbled walnuts and a dollop of Greek yoghurt on top.

Dark Chocolate Avocado Mousse

Ingredients:

- Ripe avocados

- Dark chocolate

- Maple syrup

- Vanilla extract

Instructions:

1. Smoothly combine avocados, melted dark chocolate, maple syrup, and vanilla essence.

2. Refrigerate until ready to serve.

Coconut Almond Energy Bites

Ingredients:

- Almond flour
- Shredded coconut
- Almond butter
- Dates

Instructions:

1. Combine almond flour, shredded coconut, almond butter, and dates.
2. Make bite-sized balls out of the dough.

Baked Berry Oatmeal Cups

Ingredients:

- Rolled oats
- Mixed berries
- Almond milk

- Egg

Instructions:

1. Combine the oats, berries, almond milk, and egg in a mixing bowl.
2. Bake until set in muffin cups.

Frozen Banana Bites

Ingredients:

- Bananas
- Peanut butter
- Dark chocolate
- Chopped nuts

Instructions:

1. Spread peanut butter on banana slices.
2. Dip in melted dark chocolate, then in chopped nuts.
3. Freeze until completely solid.

Greek Yogurt Parfait with Nuts and Honey

Ingredients:

- Greek yogurt
- Mixed nuts
- Honey
- Granola

Instructions:

1. Layer Greek yoghurt, mixed nuts, honey,
2. and granola.

Pumpkin Spice Muffins

Ingredients:

- Pumpkin puree
- Almond flour
- Cinnamon
- Baking powder

Instructions:

1. Combine pumpkin puree, almond flour, cinnamon, and baking powder in a mixing bowl.
2. Make muffins.

Almond Date Truffles

Ingredients:

- Almonds
- Dates
- Vanilla extract
- Shredded coconut

Instructions:

1. Combine almonds, dates, and vanilla extract in a mixing bowl.
2. Roll the mixture into truffles and roll in shredded coconut.

Berry Sorbet

Ingredients:

- Mixed berries
- Lemon juice
- Honey

Instructions:

1. Combine the berries, lemon juice, and honey in a mixing bowl.
2. Scoop and serve after freezing until firm.

Baked Pear with Cinnamon and Walnuts

Ingredients:

- Pears
- Cinnamon
- Walnuts
- Maple syrup

Instructions:

1. Slice the pears and sprinkle with cinnamon.

2. Finish with a drizzle of maple syrup and chopped walnuts.

3. Bake until the potatoes are tender.

Avocado Lime Cheesecake Bites

Ingredients:

- Avocado
- Lime
- Cream cheese
- Coconut flour

Instructions:

1. Combine avocado, lime, cream cheese, and coconut flour in a mixing bowl.

2. Refrigerate after spooning into mini muffin cups.

Cacao and Almond Butter Smoothie Bowl

Ingredients:

- Almond butter
- Cacao powder
- Banana
- Almond milk

Instructions:

1. Combine almond butter, cacao powder, banana, and almond milk in a mixing bowl.
2. Pour into a bowl and top with banana slices.

Lemon Poppy Seed Protein Balls

Ingredients:

- Protein powder
- Almond flour
- Lemon zest

- Poppy seeds

Instructions:

1. Combine protein powder, almond flour, lemon zest, and poppy seeds.
2. Make small balls out of the dough.

Berry and Mint Infused Water

Ingredients:

- Mixed berries
- Fresh mint leaves
- Water
- Ice

Instructions:

1. Infuse water with fresh mint leaves and mixed berries.
2. With ice, serve chilled.

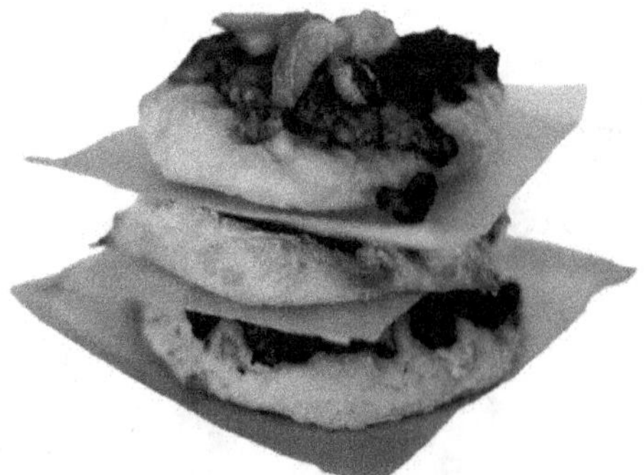

CHAPTER 5: SNACK ATTACKS

Nutty Trail Mix

Ingredients:

- Almonds
- Walnuts
- Pumpkin seeds
- Dried cranberries

Instructions:

1. Combine almonds, walnuts, pumpkin seeds, and dried cranberries.
2. Serve in snack-sized portions.

Hummus and Veggie Sticks

Ingredients:

- Chickpeas
- Tahini

- Lemon juice

- Carrot and cucumber sticks

Instructions:

1. To make hummus, combine chickpeas, tahini, and lemon juice.

2. Serve with cucumber and carrot sticks.

Greek Yogurt with Berries

Ingredients:

- Greek yogurt

- Mixed berries

- Chia seeds

- Honey

Instructions:

1. Top Greek yoghurt with berries, chia seeds,

2. and honey drizzle.

Crispy Chickpeas

Ingredients:

- Canned chickpeas
- Olive oil
- Paprika
- Sea salt

Instructions:

1. Combine chickpeas, olive oil, paprika, and sea salt in a mixing bowl.
2. Cook until crispy.

Apple Slices with Almond Butter

Ingredients:

- Apple slices
- Almond butter
- Cinnamon
- Chia seeds

Instructions:

1. On apple slices, spread almond butter.

2. Top with cinnamon and chia seeds.

Edamame and Sea Salt

Ingredients:

- Edamame beans
- Sea salt

Instructions:

1. Steam the edamame beans and season with sea salt.

Cucumber and Tzatziki Bites

Ingredients:

- Cucumber slices
- Tzatziki sauce
- Cherry tomatoes
- Fresh dill

Instructions:

1. Top cucumber slices with tzatziki, cherry tomatoes, and fresh dill.

Whole Grain Crackers with Smoked Salmon

Ingredients:

- Whole grain crackers
- Smoked salmon
- Cream cheese
- Dill

Instructions:

1. On crackers, spread cream cheese.
2. Serve with smoked salmon and dill on top.

Yogurt-Dipped Strawberries

Ingredients:

- Strawberries

- Greek yogurt

- Honey

- Crushed pistachios

Instructions:

1. Dip strawberries in Greek yoghurt.

2. Drizzle with honey and top with chopped pistachios.

Almond and Coconut Protein Balls

Ingredients:

- Almond butter

- Protein powder

- Shredded coconut

- Maple syrup

Instructions:

1. Combine almond butter, protein powder, shredded coconut, and maple syrup in a mixing bowl.

2. Make small balls out of the dough.

Carrot Cake Energy Bites

Ingredients:

- Shredded carrots
- Oats
- Cinnamon
- Almond butter

Instructions:

1. Combine shredded carrots, oats, cinnamon, and almond butter in a mixing bowl.
2. Make bite-sized balls.

Popcorn with Rosemary and Parmesan

Ingredients:

- Popped popcorn
- Olive oil

- Fresh rosemary

- Parmesan cheese

Instructions:

1. Drizzle olive oil over popcorn.

2. Sprinkle with rosemary and Parmesan cheese.

Turmeric and Ginger Tea

Ingredients:

- Turmeric tea bags

- Fresh ginger

- Lemon slices

- Honey

Instructions:

1. Make a cup of turmeric tea with fresh ginger and lemon slices.

2. Sweeten with honey.

Rice Cake with Avocado and Cherry Tomatoes

Ingredients:

- Rice cakes
- Avocado
- Cherry tomatoes
- Sea salt

Instructions:

1. On rice cakes, spread mashed avocado.
2. Sprinkle with sea salt and top with sliced cherry tomatoes.

Fruit and Nut Yogurt Parfait

Ingredients:

- Low-fat yogurt
- Mixed fruits (berries, kiwi)
- Nuts (almonds, walnuts)
- Granola

Instructions:

1. Combine low-fat yoghurt, mixed fruits, nuts,

2. and granola in a serving dish.

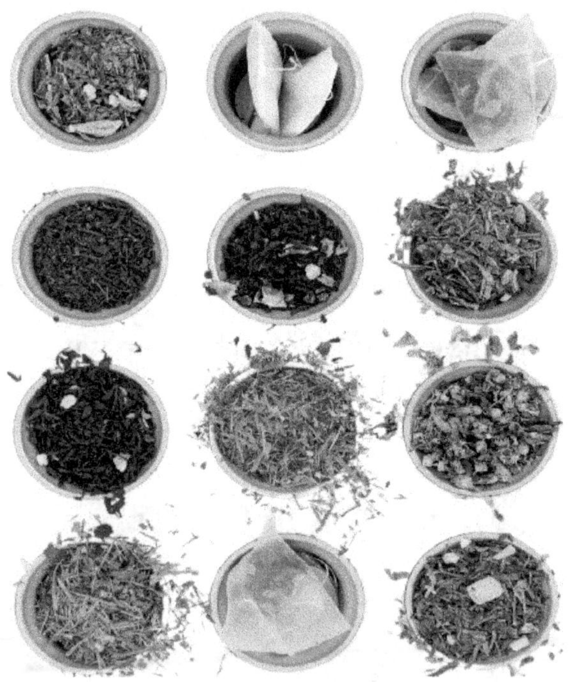

CHAPTER 6: BEVERAGES

Green Tea with Mint and Lemon

Ingredients:

- Green tea leaves
- Fresh mint leaves
- Lemon slices
- Honey (optional)

Instructions:

1. Steep green tea leaves in hot water.
2. Serve with fresh mint leaves and lemon slices.
3. If desired, add honey to taste.

Berry and Kale Smoothie

Ingredients:

- Mixed berries (blueberries, strawberries)
- Kale leaves
- Greek yogurt

- Almond milk

Instructions:

1. Blend until smooth the mixed berries, kale, Greek yoghurt, and almond milk.

Golden Milk Turmeric Latte

Ingredients:

- Turmeric powder
- Almond milk
- Cinnamon
- Ginger

Instructions:

1. Heat and stir the turmeric powder, almond milk, cinnamon,
2. and ginger until well combined.

Cucumber and Mint Infused Water

Ingredients:

- Cucumber slices
- Fresh mint leaves
- Lemon slices
- Water

Instructions:

1. In a bowl, combine cucumber slices, mint leaves, and lemon slices.
2. Refrigerate for a cool infusion.

Beet and Berry Detox Juice

Ingredients:

- Beets
- Mixed berries (raspberries, blackberries)
- Celery
- Lemon

Instructions:

1. Beet juice, mixed berries, celery and lemon.

Pomegranate Green Tea

Ingredients:

Green tea bags

- Pomegranate juice
- Fresh lime juice
- Honey (optional)

Instructions:

1. Steep green tea bags in hot water.
2. Combine pomegranate juice, fresh lime juice, and honey in a mixing bowl.

Coconut Water and Pineapple Smoothie

Ingredients:

- Coconut water
- Pineapple chunks
- Banana
- Spinach leaves

Instructions:

1. Blend until smooth the coconut water, pineapple chunks, banana, and spinach.

Chia Seed Lemonade

Ingredients:

- Lemon juice
- Chia seeds
- Agave syrup
- Water

Instructions:

1. Combine the lemon juice, chia seeds, agave syrup, and water in a mixing bowl.
2. Before serving, allow the chia seeds to expand.

Strawberry Basil Infused Water

Ingredients:

- Strawberries, sliced

- Fresh basil leaves
- Lemon slices
- Water

Instructions:

1. In a bowl, combine strawberries, basil, and lemon slices.
2. Allow it to rest for a few hours before serving.

Mango Ginger Iced Tea

Ingredients:

- Black tea bags
- Fresh mango puree
- Fresh ginger, grated
- Mint leaves

Instructions:

1. In a cup of hot water, steep two black tea bags.
2. Combine with mango puree, grated ginger, and mint leaves. Serve with ice.

Cranberry and Orange Sparkling Water

Ingredients:

- Cranberry juice (unsweetened)
- Fresh orange juice
- Sparkling water
- Ice

Instructions:

1. Combine cranberry juice and orange juice.
2. Serve over ice with sparkling water on top.

Lemon Verbena and Ginger Tea

Ingredients:

- Lemon verbena leaves
- Fresh ginger slices

- Honey (optional)
- Hot water

Instructions:

1. In a cup of hot water, steep lemon verbena leaves and fresh ginger slices.
2. If desired, add honey to taste.

Watermelon Mint Cooler

Ingredients:

- Watermelon cubes
- Fresh mint leaves
- Lime juice
- Coconut water

Instructions:

1. Combine watermelon cubes, fresh mint leaves, lime juice, and coconut water in a blender.
2. Serve over ice with a strainer.

Raspberry Hibiscus Iced Tea

Ingredients:

- Hibiscus tea bags
- Raspberries
- Mint leaves
- Agave syrup

Instructions:

1. In hot water, steep hibiscus tea bags.
2. Combine raspberries, mint leaves, and agave syrup in a mixing bowl. Chill before serving over ice.

Pineapple and Turmeric Smoothie

Ingredients:

- Pineapple chunks
- Turmeric powder
- Greek yogurt
- Almond milk

Instructions:

1. Blend until smooth the pineapple chunks, turmeric powder, Greek yoghurt, and almond milk.

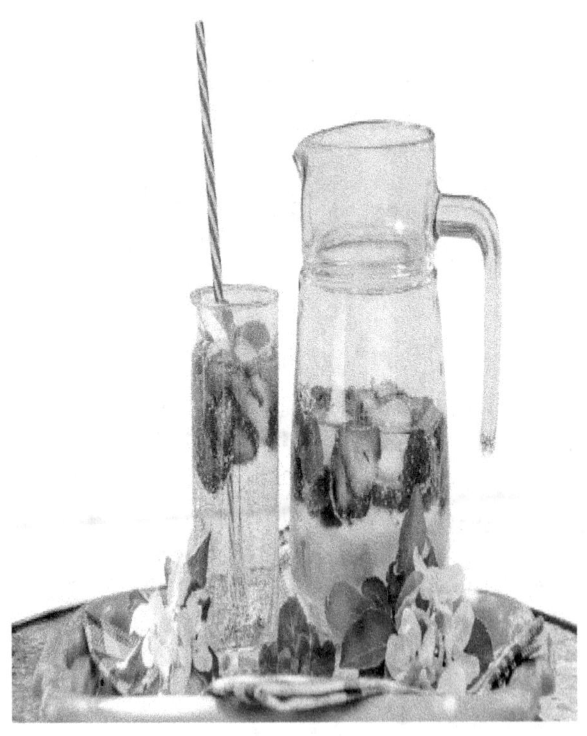

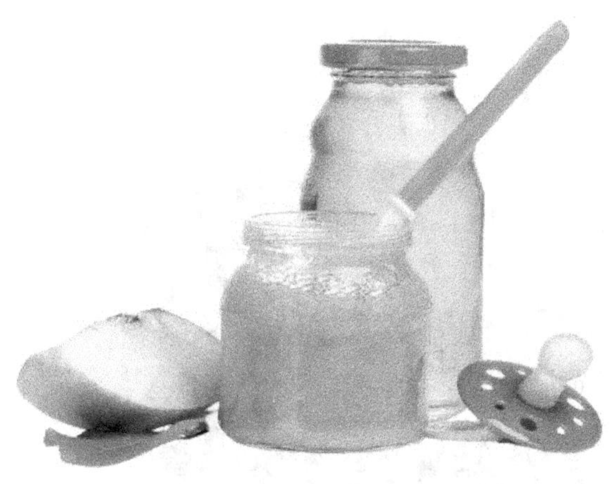

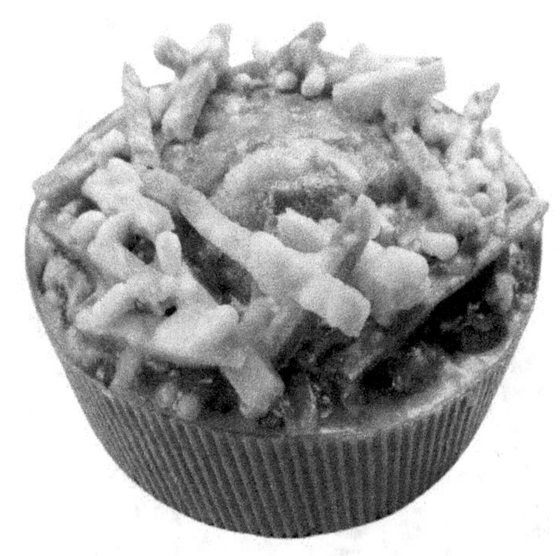

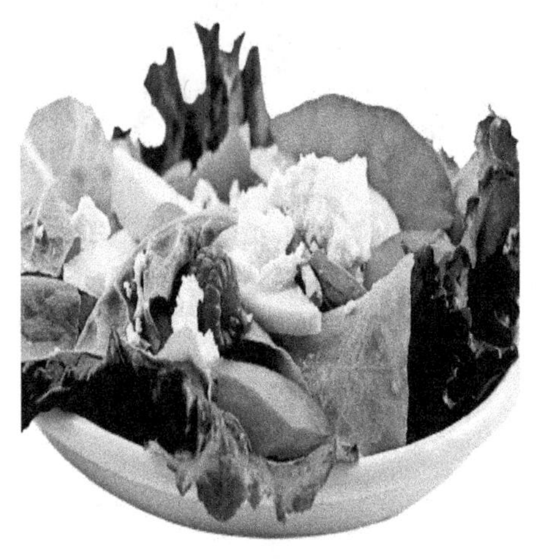

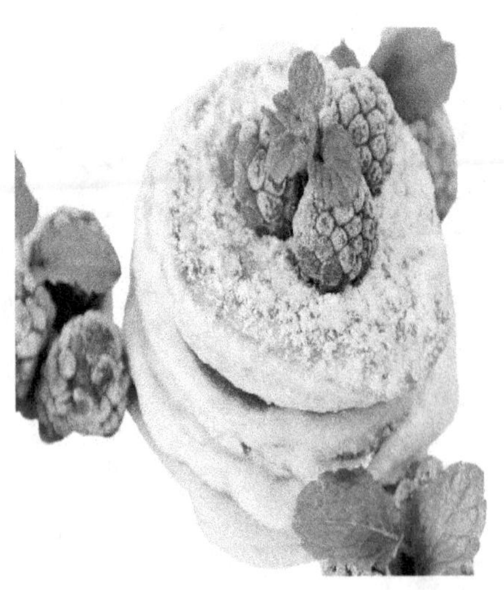

CONCLUSION

Additional Resources

Individuals navigating the challenges of breast cancer may find valuable resources to further enhance their understanding of the relationship between nutrition and well-being during this journey in addition to the Breast Cancer Diet Cookbook.

Here are some more resources:

"Anti-Cancer: A New Way of Life" by David Servan-Schreiber:

This book delves into the role of nutrition and lifestyle in cancer prevention and treatment. It provides practical advice on how to incorporate anti-cancer foods into daily meals and how to take a holistic approach to health.

Nutrition in Cancer - National Cancer Institute (NCI)

Cancer Care:

The NCI provides comprehensive information on the role of nutrition in cancer care. Their resources include guidelines, research updates, and practical tips for maintaining a healthy diet during and after cancer treatment.

American Cancer Society – Nutrition for People with Cancer:

The American Cancer Society provides a wealth of nutrition resources tailored specifically for cancer patients. Their recommendations cover topics like dealing with side effects, maintaining a healthy weight, and making informed dietary decisions.

Cancer Nutrition Consortium:

This organisation focuses on the intersection of cancer and nutrition, offering evidence-based information, webinars, and resources to people who want to improve their nutrition during and after cancer treatment.

Breastcancer.org – Nutrition and Exercise:

Breastcancer.org provides a dedicated section on nutrition and exercise, addressing common questions and concerns about diet and physical activity for breast cancer patients.

Cook for Your Life:

An online platform that provides a variety of recipes and resources for people undergoing cancer treatment. The website offers useful cooking tips and emphasises the importance of tasty and nutritious meals.

These resources supplement the Breast Cancer Diet Cookbook by providing a comprehensive understanding of how dietary choices can improve health outcomes. Individuals should seek the advice of healthcare professionals and registered dietitians to develop a personalised nutrition plan based on their specific needs and treatment protocols.